Roberta Kelly Mendonça dos Santos
Fabienne Louise Juvêncio Andrade
Fábio Correia Lima Nepomuceno

SOCIODEMOGRAPHIC AND CLINICAL PROFILE OF ELDERLY PEOPLE AT RISK OF FALLING

Roberta Kelly Mendonça dos Santos
Fabienne Louise Juvêncio Andrade
Fábio Correia Lima Nepomuceno

SOCIODEMOGRAPHIC AND CLINICAL PROFILE OF ELDERLY PEOPLE AT RISK OF FALLING

A STUDY IN PRIMARY HEALTH CARE

ScienciaScripts

Imprint

Cover image: www.ingimage.com

This book is a translation from the original published under ISBN 978-3-639-61949-2.

Publisher:
Sciencia Scripts
is a trademark of
Dodo Books Indian Ocean Ltd. and OmniScriptum S.R.L publishing group

120 High Road, East Finchley, London, N2 9ED, United Kingdom
Str. Armeneasca 28/1, office 1, Chisinau MD-2012, Republic of Moldova, Europe
Managing Directors: Ieva Konstantinova, Victoria Ursu
info@omniscriptum.com

Printed at: see last page
ISBN: 978-620-8-51677-2

CONTENTS

INTRODUCTION 4
CHAPTER 1- METHODOLOGICAL ASPECTS 7
CHAPTER 2- SOCIO-DEMOGRAPHIC AND CLINICAL DATA COLLECTION INSTRUMENTS 8
CHAPTER 3- STATISTICAL ANALYSIS 29
CHAPTER 4- RESULTS 31
CHAPTER 5- PROFILE OF COMMUNITY-DWELLING ELDERLY AT RISK OF FALLING 39
REFERENCES 46

SOCIODEMOGRAPHIC AND CLINICAL PROFILE OF ELDERLY PEOPLE AT RISK OF FALLING: A PRIMARY HEALTH CARE STUDY

Population ageing is one of society's most significant events and over the years it has become increasingly significant, particularly in developing countries. In Brazil, the population segment represented by the elderly is the fastest growing, and by 2050, projections suggest that 30 per cent of Brazilians will be represented by people aged 60 or over, at which point the country will rank sixth among those with the highest number of elderly people. At the same time as demographic changes, there are changes in morbidity and mortality patterns characterised by an increase in chronic degenerative diseases and factors that can result in dependency and a lower quality of life, particularly falls. In addition to its debilitating nature, falls are important in the public health scenario due to their high prevalence, which burdens the health system as the demand for medical and hospital care to treat associated injuries increases. There is still a need for studies on the factors associated with falls in primary care, given the growing number of elderly people assisted by the Family Health Strategy (ESF) and the need for preventive policies that take into account the specific characteristics and demands of each society.

SUMMARY

The high incidence of falls in the elderly, associated with high morbidity and mortality and the increased economic costs of treating injuries, make this a public health problem, signalling the need to seek preventive strategies based on knowledge of the population's main characteristics and needs. Despite the fact that studies have reported aspects related to the risk of falling, there is a need to study the factors associated with falls in community-dwelling elderly people, within the logic of primary care and the Family Health Strategy, considering the specific characteristics and demands of the people assigned to the UBS.The aim of this study is to analyse the prevalence and factors associated with falls in elderly people assigned to a Basic Health Unit (UBS) in the municipality of Natal/RN. This is a cross-sectional study of 280 elderly people whose data was collected on the premises of the BHU. The association between the outcomes falls and recurrent falls and the independent variables was verified using bivariate analysis and Poisson regression, with calculation of the respective prevalence ratios. The elderly were predominantly female (68.2%), with a mean age of 71.6 years (± 6.7), literate (54.6%), not retired (73.5%) and sedentary (87.1%). 53.6 per cent of the elderly fell, but 27.8 per cent fell twice or more. The predictive model for falls included female gender (PR= 1.81), presence of osteoarticular diseases (PR= 1.71) and balance impairment (PR= 0.88), while functional mobility (PR= 0.94), fear of falling (PR= 1.21) and balance deficit (PR= 0.80) made up the final model for recurrent falls. There was a higher prevalence of a single episode of falling and the associated factors included socio-demographic, health and physical performance variables. On the other hand, only physical performance variables were associated with the occurrence of two or more falls.

Keywords: Ageing, Falls, Risk Factors, Basic Health Unit, Primary Care.

INTRODUCTION

The progressive reduction in the fertility rate associated with the increase in life expectancy resulting from improvements in health care has resulted in the ageing of the world population, which opens up discussion about disabling events in this age group, highlighting the occurrence of falls due to their physical, psychological, social and health system consequences (ESCORSIM, 2021).

A fall is defined as an unintentional displacement of the body to a level lower than the initial position that results from the individual's inability to correct this displacement in a timely manner, and is determined by multifactorial circumstances that compromise stability. Its prevalence is associated with advancing age, which makes falls a public health problem due to their increasing frequency, which accompanies the increase in the number of elderly people in the world (GONÇALVES et al., 2022).

Population studies indicate that 30% to 60% of elderly people living in communities fall every year. In Brazil, around 30% of people aged 65 or over fall at least once a year and of these, 13% become recurrent fallers (NASCIMENTO et al., 2008).

Despite the frequency with which they occur, falls have consequences both for health services in terms of the use of resources and the occupation of hospital beds, and for the individual, in terms of loss of functional capacity, autonomy and independence, psychological trauma and even the risk of death (PAIVA et al.,

2019).

In addition to the individual repercussions, data from the Ministry of Health show that in 2006, the Unified Health System (SUS) spent R$49 million on hospital admissions of elderly people due to hip fractures caused by falls, with this figure rising to R$57.6 million in 2009 (LABOISSIÈRE, 2010).

Given the above, it can be understood that the occurrence of falls has an impact not only on the lives of the elderly, but also demands high financial costs for the Brazilian state, highlighting the need for studies that analyse the main causes and factors associated with the risk of falling in community-dwelling elderly people, in order to build preventive strategies based on the specific demands of each population (CRUZ; LEITE, 2018).

Although the prevention of falls is provided for in primary preventive services aimed at maintaining the health of elderly Brazilians, public health actions still do not incorporate specific interventions for the problem in question. Studies have investigated the causes that lead older people to fall, but there is still a need for research in primary care, given the growing number of older people who benefit from the assistance offered by the Family Health Strategy (ESF) and the need for preventive policies that take into account the particularities and specific demands of societies. In this scenario, health teams appear as allies by fulfilling their role in identifying the most common risk situations to which the elderly are exposed, as well as devising strategies to deal with them (PINHO et al., 2012).

Among the skills and duties of the primary care team under the UBS strategy, we highlight the development of both collective and individual actions aimed at maintaining the maximum independence, functionality and autonomy of the elderly, as well as encouraging community participation in health education practices for these individuals. These actions can be developed more rigorously within the ESF, given that the team is able to carefully identify the real needs of the population it assists (CRUZ; LEITE, 2018).

The aim of this study was to analyse the sociodemographic and clinical profile of elderly people at risk of falling, who live in the community and are affiliated to a Basic Health Unit (BHU) in the municipality of Natal.

CHAPTER 1 - METHODOLOGICAL ASPECTS

The design of this study complied with the recommendations of STROBE (*Strengthening the Reporting of Observational Studies in Epidemiology*) for observational *studies*. This is a descriptive cross-sectional epidemiological study carried out with 280 elderly users registered at the Felipe Camarão II UBS, located in the Felipe Camarão neighbourhood in the city of Natal, RN. It is a low economic class neighbourhood, located in the west of the municipality, with a land area of 663.40 ha and a population of approximately 50,997 inhabitants, representing 6.37% of the city's population, making it the third most populous neighbourhood in the municipality .·

The Felipe Camarão BHU is home to four extended ESF teams that provide assistance to approximately 4,000 families, covering around 15,000 residents.

The study population was made up of all the elderly people registered at the above-mentioned UBS (n=747). However, the medical records and the health team were initially consulted to choose the volunteers who would be able to take part in the study according to the inclusion criteria. In order to be included, the volunteers had to be aged 60 or over, not need help from others to carry out basic activities of daily living, such as feeding, bathing, dressing and walking, not use walking aids and not have any illness, health problem and/or visual, hearing or other impairment that would compromise communication or the performance of the tests in the assessment.

CHAPTER 2- SOCIO-DEMOGRAPHIC AND CLINICAL DATA COLLECTION INSTRUMENTS

Data was collected on the premises of the UBS between March and August 2012, always by the same researcher who carried out an assessment comprising a questionnaire containing socio-demographic information (age, gender, marital status, physical activity), self-reported health information, scales and tests validated in the Brazilian version for assessing physical and psychosocial performance in the elderly, as well as recording the occurrence of falls and recurrent falls.

The history of falls was recorded by asking the person if they had fallen in the 12 months prior to the survey. To do this, a retrospective evaluation was carried out in which the person being analysed had to remember the number of falls they had suffered in the last year: no falls, one fall, or two or more falls.

Health conditions were recorded by asking about the presence of visual impairment, Systemic Arterial Hypertension (SAH), Osteoarticular Disease (OAD), Diabetes Mellitus (DM), heart disease and comorbidity, i.e. the association of at least two of these pathologies or others in the same individual.

2.1 Evaluation procedures

The elderly were invited by the CHAs to come individually to a UBS in Natal, on a scheduled date and time, so that the assessment procedures could begin. The figure below shows the Basic Health Unit where the study was carried out.

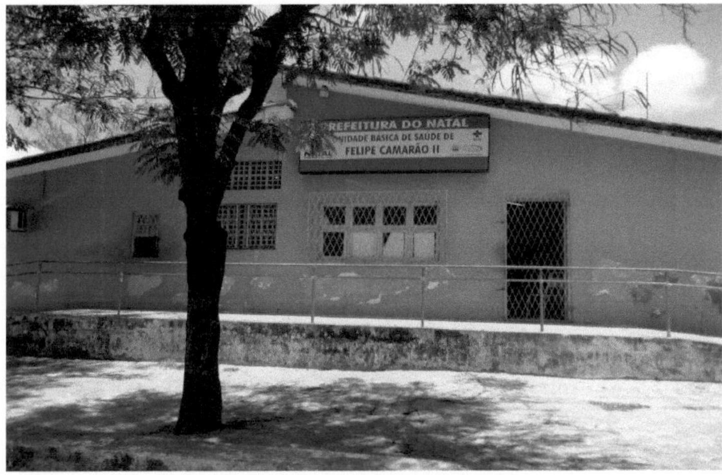

Figure 1- Felipe Camarão Basic Health Unit, where the study was carried out

After receiving the appropriate guidance on the objectives of the study, the volunteers underwent an initial assessment, where information regarding the inclusion criteria was collected, in addition to analysing the following outcome measures: (1) BSE; (2) TUGT; (3) FES-I-Brazil.

A) Berg Balance Scale (BBS)

The BBS is a widely used instrument for assessing static and dynamic functional balance in the elderly because it is low cost, easy and quick to apply, and has intra- and inter-observer reliability of 0.98. This study used the Brazilian version translated and adapted by Miyamoto et al (2004).

The BSE is made up of 14 tasks representative of ADLs, such as sitting, standing, leaning forward, turning round and looking back, picking up an object from the floor, among others. Each item on the scale is made up of 5 alternatives whose scores range from 0 to 4 points, with zero indicating the inability to perform the task and four indicating the ability to perform it. The total score can vary from 0 to 56 points, with the higher value representing better performance in the test and therefore better balance (WHITNEY, 1998).

The BSE was used not only as an outcome measure to analyse the effectiveness of the interventions, but also as an inclusion criterion, with 52 being the cut-off point for the subject to take part in the research (SILSUPADOL, 2009).

B) Timed Up and Go Test (TUGT)

The TUGT is a test used to assess an individual's functional mobility by analysing sitting balance, transfers from sitting to standing, walking stability and gait changes without the use of compensatory strategies (SHUMWAY-COOK, 2008).

The test quantifies functional mobility in seconds through the time it takes the individual to perform the task, i.e. in how many seconds the volunteer gets up from a standardised chair approximately 46 centimetres high with armrests, walks 3 metres, turns around, walks back to the chair and sits down again (PODSIADLO; RICHARDSON, 1991).

At the start of the test, the elderly person was seated with their back against the back of the chair and at the end they had to lean back again. The volunteer was given the command "go" to perform the test and the time was timed from the moment the command was given until the moment they sat down and leaned back on the chair. The test was carried out twice, once for familiarisation and once to record the measurement.

Among healthy adults, the average time taken to complete the test is 10 seconds. According to Shumway-Cook et al. (2008), elderly people who complete the TUGT in less than 20 seconds are considered independent in their ADLs and have sufficient walking speed to get around in the community. Those who complete the task in more than 13.5 seconds are at greater risk of falls.

C) International Falls Effectiveness Scale Brazil (FES-I-Brazil)

The International Falls Efficacy Scale Brazil assesses the fear of falling through questions that analyse how worried the individual is about the possibility of suffering a fall if they were to perform certain tasks. It is an instrument based on excellent psychometric properties for the Brazilian population, which was validated and adapted from the *Falls Efficacy Scale - International* (FES-I) (YARDLEY et al., 2005).

Fear of falling is assessed in 16 different daily activities, with values ranging from 16 points for people with no concern about falling to 64 points for those with extreme concern (CAMARGO et al., 2010; LOPRES et al., 2009).

The FES-I score was recorded when the questionnaire was applied. To do this, the elderly person was asked to imagine themselves carrying out the activities proposed by the scale and then mention their level of concern about falling: not at all concerned, a little concerned or extremely concerned.

Below are the forms used to collect the survey data.

FIRST PHASE OF EVALUATION - Inclusion Criteria

I. PERSONAL DATA:

Name:..

..

Individual no:.. Sex: F ( ) M

( )

Date of birth:..../..../.... Age:...

Address:..

Contact telephone

numbers:../ ....

Marital status:.......................................

Education:...

Profession:..Occupation:.......................

....

II. ANTHROPOMETRIC MEASUREMENTS:

Height(cm)...Weight(kg):..........

....

BMI

(weight/(height)^2:...

III. CLINICAL DATA:

Presence of pathologies

( ) Systemic Arterial Hypertension ( ) Respiratory Diseases

( ) Diabetes Mellitus ( ) Rheumatic Diseases

( ) Neurological Disorders ( ) Cardiac Diseases

( ) Orthopaedic disorders

( ) Hearing disorders Corrected ( )Yes ( )No

( ) Visual disturbances Corrected ( ) Yes ( )No

( ) Other:..

Do you need help with ADLs: ( ) Yes ( ) No

What

activity(ies):...

...

Do you use walking aids: ( ) Yes ( ) No

Which:...

.....

Do you use continuous medication: ( ) Yes ( ) No

Which

ones:...

.

Vital Signs:

P.A.:..FC:...FR:.............

...

IV. BERG EQUILIBRIUM SCALE (EEB)

1. From sitting to standing.

Instruction: Please stand up and try not to use your hands as support.

Graduation: Please tick the lowest category that applies

(4) can stand up without the help of their hands and can stabilise themselves.

(3) stands on their own using their hands.

(2) stands up using his hands after numerous attempts.

(1) needs minimal help to stand or stabilise themselves.

(0) needs maximum or moderate help to stand.

2. Standing without support.

Instruction: Stand for two minutes without holding on.

Graduation: Please tick the lowest category that applies

(4) Stand safely for two minutes.

(3) Stand for two minutes with supervision.

(2) Stand for 30 seconds without support.

(1) Makes numerous attempts to stand for 30 seconds without support.

(0) Unable to stand for 30 seconds without support.

NOTE: If the individual is able to stand for 2 minutes safely, score the maximum category for sitting without support. Go on to change position from standing to sitting.

3. Sitting with feet flat on the floor.

Instructions: Sit with your arms crossed for 2 minutes.

Graduation: Please tick the lowest category that applies

(4) sit securely and firmly for 2 minutes.

(3) sits for 2 minutes under supervision.

(2) sit for 30 seconds.

(1) sit for 10 seconds.

(0) unable to sit for 10 seconds without support.

4. From standing to sitting.

Instruction: Please sit down.

Graduation: Please tick the lowest category that applies

(4) Sits safely with minimal use of hands.

(3) Control the descent using your hands.

(2) Use the back of your leg against the chair to control the descent.

(1) Sits independently, but slumps uncontrollably.

(0) needs help to sit up.

5. Transfers.

Instruction: Please move from the chair to the bed and back to the chair again. In one direction, a seat with an armrest and in the other direction a seat without an armrest.

Graduation: Please tick the lowest category that applies

(4) Transfer carefully, with minimal use of hands.

(3) Transfers carefully and requires the use of hands.

(2) Transfers with verbal cues and/or supervision.

(1) needs someone to help.

(0) Needs two people for help or supervision for safety.

6. Standing, without support and eyes closed.

Instruction: Close your eyes and stay still for 10 seconds.

Graduation: Please tick the lowest category that applies

(4) Stand safely for 10 seconds.

(3) Stand for 10 seconds with supervision.

(2) Stand for 3 seconds.

(1) Unable to stand for 3 seconds, but remains immobile.

(0) Needs help to avoid falling.

7. Standing without support with feet together.

Instructions: Put your feet together and stand up straight.

Graduation: Please tick the lowest category that applies

(4) Put your feet together independently and stay safely for 1 minute.

(3) Put your feet together independently and stay for 1 minute With supervision.

(2) Places the feet together independently, but is unable to hold them together for 30 seconds.

(1) Needs help to get into position, but can hold it for 15 seconds. with feet together.

(0) Needs help to get into position and unable to hold it for 15 seconds.

The following items will be carried out while the individual is standing without support.

8. Reach forwards with arms outstretched.

Instructions: Raise your arms to 90□. Lengthen your fingers and reach forwards as far as you can (the examiner should place a ruler at the end of your fingertips when your arms are at 90□. Your fingers should not touch the ruler while you are reaching forwards. The measurement taken is the distance forwards that the fingers reach when the individual is at their maximum forward lean).

Graduation: Please tick the lowest category that applies

(4) Safely reaches forwards > 10 inches (25.4 cm).

(3) Safely reaches forwards > 5 inches (12.7 cm).

(2) Safely reaches forwards > 2 inches (5.08 cm).

(1) Reaches ahead, but needs supervision.

(0) Needs help to avoid falling.

9. Pick up an object from the floor.

Instruction: Pick up the shoe or slipper in front of your feet.

Graduation: Please tick the lowest category that applies

(4) Easily and safely picks up the shoe.

(3) Can pick up the shoe, but needs supervision.

(2) Unable to pick up the shoe, but reaches 1-2 inches (2.54-5.05 cm) from the shoe and maintains balance independently.

(1) Unable to pick up and needs supervision while trying.

(0) Unable to try / needs supervision to avoid falling.

10. Turning to look back/over right and left shoulders.

Instruction: Turn round to look back over your left shoulder. Now repeat for the right.

Graduation: Please tick the lowest category that applies

(4) Looks back from both sides with good weight transfer.

(3) Look back from one side only, the other side shows less weight transfer.

(2) Turn to one side only, but keep your balance.

(1) Needs supervision when turning round.

(0) Needs supervision to avoid falling.

11. Turn 360□.

Instructions: Turn completely around yourself making a full circle. Pause. Now turn in a complete circle in the other direction.

Graduation: Please tick the lowest category that applies

(4) Turn 360□ safely in less than 4 seconds each way.

(3) Turn 360□ safely to one side in less than 4 seconds.

(2) Turn 360□ safely, but slowly.

(1) Needs close supervision or verbal cues

(0) Needs help while turning.

Dynamic weight transfer while standing without support.

12. Playing a stool.

Instructions: Place each foot alternately on the stool. Continue until each foot has touched the stool 4 times.

Graduation: Please tick the lowest category that applies

(4) Able to stand independently and safely and complete 8 touches in 20 seconds .

(3) Able to stand independently and complete 8 touches in more than 20 seconds.

(2) Able to complete 4 rings unaided and with supervision.

(1) Able to complete more than 2 touches and needs minimal help.

(0) Needs help to avoid falling/unable to try.

13. Stand without support with one foot in front.

Instruction: (demonstrate to the subject) Place one foot directly in front of the other. If you feel you can't place your foot directly in front of the other, try stepping forwards, far enough so that the heel of your front foot is in front of the toes of the other foot.

Graduation: Please tick the lowest category that applies

(4) able to position the foot well forward independently and stay there for 30 seconds.

(3) able to position one foot in front of the other independently and remain there for 30 seconds.

(2) able to take a small step independently and stay there for 30 seconds.

(1) needs help to take the step, but can stay for 15 seconds.

(0) loses balance when taking a step or standing up.

14. Stand on one leg.

Instructions: Stand on one leg for as long as you can without holding on.

Graduation: Please tick the lowest category that applies

(4) able to raise the leg independently and stay for more than 10 seconds.

(3) able to raise the leg independently and stay for 5 - 10 seconds.

(2) able to raise the leg independently and remain for a period of 3 seconds or more.

(1) tries to lift leg; unable to maintain for 3 seconds, but continues to stand independently.

(0) unable to try or needs assistance to prevent a fall.

TOTAL SCORE: _________/ 56 points.

After going through the initial assessment procedure, analysing the inclusion criteria, the eligible elderly were submitted to the second assessment stage, as follows.

SECOND STAGE OF EVALUATION-Outcome Measures
I. **TIMED UP and GO TEST** (PODSIADLO; RICHARDSON, 1991) **Instructions**: the subject is seated in a chair approximately 45 cm high, with armrests, with their back supported, wearing their usual footwear and/or walking aids. After the command "go", the subject must get up from the chair and walk a linear distance of 3 metres, with safe steps, return to the chair and sit down again. **Time spent on the task**: ___s. II. **FALLS EFFICACY SCALE INTERNACIONAL-BRASIL (FES- I-BRASIL)** **Now we'd like to ask you a few questions about your concerns regarding the possibility of falling. Please answer by imagining how you normally do the activity. If you don't currently do the activity (e.g. someone goes shopping for you), answer in a way that shows how you would feel about falling if you had to do that activity. For each of the following activities, please tick the box that most closely matches your opinion of how worried you would be about falling if you did this activity.**

		Not one little worried 1	**A little worried 2**	**A lot worried 3**	**Extremely worried 4**
1	Cleaning the house (e.g: wipe, vacuum or dusting).	1	2	3	4
2	Putting on or taking off clothes.	1	2	3	4
3	Preparing meals simple.	1	2	3	4
4	To	bathing . 1	2	3	4
5	Shopping.	1	2	3	4
6	Sitting or getting up from a chair.	1	2	3	4
7	Up or down	1	2	3	4

	stairs.				
8	Walking through vizi	hance. 1	2	3	4
9	Taking something from above of your head or c	sion. 1	2	3	4
1	Going to answer the phone before it stops play.	1	2	3	4
11	Walking on slippery surface (e.g. wet floor).	1	2	3	4
	2 Visiting a friend or relative	1	2	3	4
13	Walking in places full of people.	1	2	3	4
14	Walking on uneven surface (with stones,	1	2	3	4

	bumpy).				
15	Up or down a slope.	1	2	3	4
16	Going to an activity social (e.g. religious act, family reunion or meeting at the club).	1	2	3	4

III. HISTORY OF FALLS

1. Have you suffered a fall(s) in the last year?

   ( ) no falls ( ) 1 fall ( ) 2 or more falls

2. Crash site:

   ( ) at home ( ) away from home

3. Did you need help getting up?

   ( ) yes ( ) no

4. Did the fall result in injury?

   ( ) yes ( ) no Which?______________________

5. Have you restricted your usual activities because of the fall?

   ( ) yes ( ) no Which one(s)?____________________

6. If you have restricted it, for what reason?

   ( ) fear ( ) pain ( ) difficulty walking ( ) other _____

7. What is the mechanism of the fall?

   ( ) fell to one side ( ) fell backwards ( ) fell forwards

   ( ) fell to his knees

8. What was the circumstance?

   ( ) tripped ( ) slipped

   ( ) fainted ( ) lost his balance

   ( ) sudden weakness ( ) darkening of vision

   ( ) loss of attention ( ) pain/site:___________________

   ( ) dizziness or vertigo ( ) other _____________________

9. Have you changed or increased any medication?

   ( ) yes/ which? ______________________ ( ) no

10. Almost falling?

    ( ) yes ( ) no

CHAPTER 3- STATISTICAL ANALYSIS

The data was analysed using the *Statistical Package for the Social Sciences* ® (SPSS) *software* version 17.0, with a significance level of 5% ($p<0.05$). Descriptive statistics were carried out using distribution measures (mean, standard deviation - SD, absolute and relative frequency), considering the variables of interest in order to characterise the sample.

In the analytical approach, bivariate analysis was initially carried out using Pearson's chi-squared test to check for associations between categorical variables and the t-test for independent samples to compare means between groups, considering that all the data had a normal distribution according to the Komolgorov-Sminorv (K-S) test.

The Poisson Regression model was then used to identify the possible independent variables associated with the outcomes, calculating the respective prevalence ratios (PR). The outcome used was the occurrence of falls and recurrent falls in the year prior to the study and the variables tested in the models were: gender, age group, marital status, schooling, physical activity, being retired or not, self-reported presence of pathologies and comorbidities, as well as the use of continuous medication and psychotropic drugs.

This study was submitted to the Research Ethics Committee of the Federal University of Rio Grande do Norte, in accordance with Resolution 196/96 of the

National Health Council, and was approved. All participants received clarification and detailed information about the objectives of the study and the procedures to which they would be subjected, and signed the Free and Informed Consent Form.

CHAPTER 4- RESULTS

Considering the established inclusion criteria, 464 elderly users were included in the study and distributed among the Community Health Agents (CHAs) in their respective catchment areas to be called in for the assessment. Of these, 12 had moved house, 27 could not be found on three consecutive visits made on different days and at different times, 24 said they could not be absent from work as they worked both days, 12 had died, 66 did not attend the assessment, 29 refused to take part in the study and 14 were not invited by the CHAs. All these elderly people were therefore excluded from the study so that 280 volunteers were assessed, making up the final sample.

The picture below shows the multidisciplinary team meeting with a group of elderly people to explain the objectives and stages of the study.

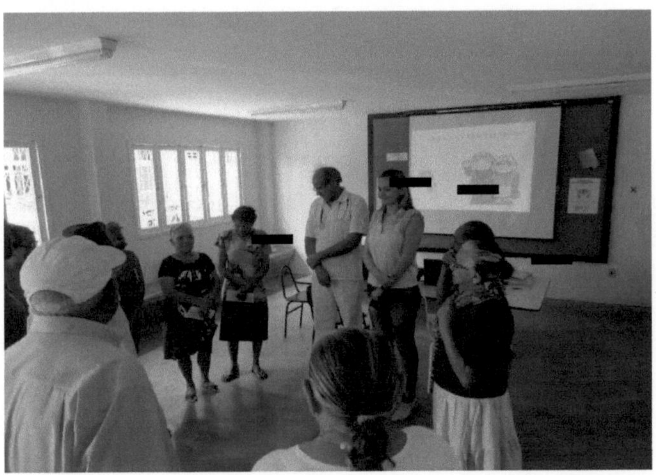

Figure 2 - Meeting with the multidisciplinary team to explain the objectives and procedures of the study.

Of the 280 elderly people studied, 68.2% were female and the majority were aged 70 or over (57.8%), with an average age of 71.6 (± 6.7) years. The prevalence of at least one episode of falling was 53.6%, and the majority of those who fell were women (74.6%).

Table 1 shows the description of the sample and the distribution of elderly people who fell or not according to socio-demographic and health characteristics. It was found that 141 (50.3%) volunteers were married, 153 (54.6%) were literate, 206 (73.6%) were still working and 244 (87.1%) did not practice any type of physical activity. When asked about their state of health, 131 (46.8%) said they had comorbidities, with visual impairment being the most prevalent pathology (68.2%). Most of the elderly reported using continuous medication (69%).

The independent variables gender, presence of comorbidity, osteoarticular disease and diabetes mellitus were significantly associated with the outcome fall in the last year.

Table 1. Occurrence of falls and associated factors according to socio-demographic and health-related variables of the elderly. Natal, RN, 2012.

Variables		Fall in the last year		
		No	Yes	p-value
Age n (%)	60 to 69 years old	53 (40,8)	65 (44,0)	0,66
	over 69	77 (59,2)	85 (56,0)	
Sex n (%)	Male	51 (39,2)	38 (25,3)	0,01
	Female	79 (60,8)	112 (74,7)	

Marital status n (%)	Single/divorced/widowed	68 (52,3)	71 (47,3)	0,40
	Married/in a stable union	62 (47,7)	79 (52,7)	
Schooling n (%)	Not literate	61 (47,0)	66 (44,0)	0,62
	Literate	69 (53,0)	84 (56,0)	
Physical Activity n (%)	No	113 (86,9)	131 (87,3)	0,91
	Yes	17 (13,1)	19 (12,7)	
Retired n (%)	No	99 (76,1)	107 (71,3)	0,36
	Yes	31 (23,8)	43 (28,7)	
Comorbidities n (%)	No	70 (53,8)	61 (40,7)	0,02
	Yes	60 (46,1)	89 (59,3)	
Visual impairment n (%)	No	44 (33,8)	45 (30,0)	0,49
	Yes	86 (66,2)	105 (70,0)	
Hypertension n (%)	No	43 (33,1)	55 (36,7)	0,53
	Yes	87 (66,9)	95 (63,3)	
Osteoarticular disease n (%)	No	65 (50,0)	56 (37,3)	0,03
	Yes	65 (50,0)	94 (62,7)	
Diabetes Mellitus n (%)	No	105 (80,8)	104 (69,3)	0,02
	Yes	25 (19,2)	46 (30,7)	
Heart disease n (%)	No	113 (86,9)	124 (82,7)	0,32
	Yes	17 (13,1)	26 (17,3)	
Use of Continuous Medication n (%)	No	42 (32,3)	45 (30,0)	0,69
	Yes	88 (67,7)	105 (70,0)	
Use of Psychotropic Medication n(%)	No	122 (93,8)	133 (88,7)	0,13
	Yes	8 (6,2)	17 (11,3)	

Figure 3 shows the frequency of falls among the elderly people assessed.

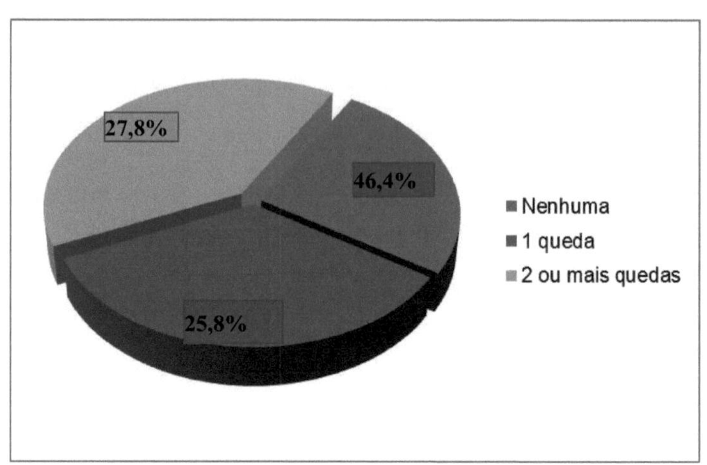

Figure 3- Prevalence of falls and recurrent falls

Table 2 shows the characteristics of the elderly with a record of recurrent falls. Of the volunteers assessed, 27.8 per cent had two or more episodes of falling, and the majority were female (80.7 per cent). Female gender (p< 0.01) and self-reported osteoarticular disease (p< 0.01) were associated with this variable.

Table 2. Occurrence of recurrent falls and associated factors according to socio-demographic and health-related variables of the elderly. Natal, RN, 2012.

Variables		Recurrent falls				
		No		Yes		p-value
Age n (%)	60 to 69 years old	83	(41,1)	35	(44,9)	0,56
	Over 69 years old	119	(58,9)	43	(55,1)	
Sex n (%)	Male	74	(36,6)	15	(19,2)	< 0,01
	Female	128	(63,3)	63	(80,8)	
Marital status n (%)	Single/divorced/widowed	100	(49,5)	39	(50,0)	0,94
	Married/in a stable union	102	(50,5)	39	(50,0)	
Schooling n (%)	Not literate	88	(43,6)	39	(50,0)	0,33
	Literate	114	(56,4)	39	(50,0)	

Practising Physical Activity n (%)				0,99
	No	175 (94,6)	69 (72,6)	
	Yes	10 (5,4)	26 (27,3)	
Retired n (%)				0,85
	No	148 (73,2)	58 (74,3)	
	Yes	54 (26,7)	20 (25,6)	
Comorbidities n (%)				0,08
	No	101 (50,0)	48 (61,5)	
	Yes	101 (50,0)	30 (38,4)	
Visual impairment n (%)				0,17
	No	133 (65,8)	58 (74,3)	
	Yes	69 (34,1)	20 (25,6)	
Hypertension n (%)				0,63
	No	133 (65,8)	49 (62,8)	
	Yes	69 (34,1)	29 (37,1)	
Osteoarticular disease n (%)				< 0,01
	No	105 (51,9)	51 (65,4)	
	Yes	97 (48,0)	27 (34,6)	
Diabetes Mellitus n (%)				0,11
	No	46 (22,8)	25 (32,0)	
	Yes	156 (77,2)	53 (68,0)	
Heart disease n (%)				0,45
	No	29 (14,3)	14 (17,9)	
	Yes	173 (85,6)	64 (82,0)	
Use of Continuous Medication n (%)				0,35
	No	136 (67,3)	57 (73,1)	
	Yes	66 (32,6)	21 (26,9)	
Use of Psychotropic Medication n (%)				0,15
	No	15 (7,4)	10 (12,8)	
	Yes	187 (92,6)	68 (87,2)	

With regard to the physical and psychosocial performance variables, table 3 shows that the elderly with a record of falls had lower performance in activities involving functional balance assessed by the BSE ($p< 0.01$), as well as lower self-efficacy in preventing falls ($p< 0.01$). For recurrent falls, there was a statistically significant difference in the means obtained in all the physical performance variables, so that the elderly who fell twice or more showed lower performance in the scores obtained in the BSE ($p< 0.01$), TUG ($p= 0.03$), FES - I ($p< 0.01$) and MMSE ($p= 0.03$).

The variables selected to build the final model of falls and recurrent falls using multiple logistic regression analysis are described in Table 4. After adjusting for the independent variables, female gender ($PR_{adjusted} = 1.81$), self-reported osteoarticular disease ($PR_{adjusted} = 1.71$) and poor performance in the activities assessed by the BSE ($PR_{adjusted} = 0.88$) remained directly associated with the occurrence of falls.

Table 3. Analysis of the physical and psychosocial performance variables of the elderly with and without a record of falls and recurrent falls in the year prior to the survey. Natal, RN, 2012.

Variables	**Fall**			**Recurring fall**		
	Yes	**No**	**p-value**	**Yes**	**No**	**p-value**
BSE, μ (SD)	49,9 (±5,61)	52,9 (±3,11)	< 0,01	49,4 (±4,74)	51,7 (±5,24)	< 0,01
TUG, μ (SD)	15,4 (±6,32)	13,9 (±8,28)	0,10	16,2 (±7,56)	14,1 (±7,15)	0,03

FES - I, μ (SD)	32,5 (±10,67)	26,8 (±9,67)	< 0,01	34,5 (±10,02)	28,3 (±10,44)	< 0,01
MMSE, μ (SD)	20,9 (±4,93)	21,36(±3,46)	0,38	20,2 (±4,28)	21,4 (±4,31)	0,03

With regard to recurrent falls, it was observed that low scores on the BBS and TUG were risk factors for the condition, since the values obtained were, respectively, BBS ($PR_{adjusted=}$ 0.08) and TUG ($PR_{adjusted=}$ 0.94). With regard to the fear of falling, the analysis shows that the absence of fear was a protective factor for the event in question ($PR_{adjusted=}$ 1.21).

Table 4 - Final model of the association between the variables analysed and the occurrence of falls and recurrent falls. Natal, RN, 2013.

Variables	Fall		Recurring fall	
	Adjusted PR (95%	Valorp	Adjusted PR (95%	Valorp
Sex			--	--
Male	1			
Female	1, 81 (1,21 - 2,67)	0,03		
DOA			--	--
No	1			
Yes	1, 71 (1,10 - 3,09)	0,03		
BBS	0,88 (0,77 - 0,96)	< 0,01	0, 80 (0,75 - 0,85)	0,03
FES - I	--	--	1, 21 (1,12 - 1,31)	0,02
TUG	--	--	0, 94 (0,85 - 0,98)	0,01

BBS = Berg Balance Scale; TUG = Tumed Up and Go; FES - I = International Falls Effectiveness Scale; MMSE = Mini Mental State Examination.

CHAPTER 5- PROFILE OF COMMUNITY-DWELLING ELDERLY AT RISK OF FALLING

The sociodemographic profile of the elderly studied is similar to that found in Brazilian studies involving community elderly people assisted by the UBS, showing a sample of predominantly female, literate, married, sedentary individuals, with an accumulation of self-reported diagnoses and use of continuous medication (CRUz et al., 2012; DANTAS et al., 2012).

The majority of the sample was made up of women, which is consistent with data shown in studies in which group approaches within the UBS have attracted a strong female presence. Bertakis et al. (2000) explain that women seek preventive health services more often than men, and that this is associated with their reproductive biology, difference in health perception and the high morbidity rate among them.

A striking feature of this study is the low level of schooling, since 31.4% of the volunteers have never been to school and 57.1% have incomplete primary education. The large number of elderly people who live in the community and have a low level of education has also been identified in other studies, which is an important risk factor for falling. There is an association between low levels of education and falls. People with a higher level of education have healthier habits, are more concerned about their health and their ability to recover, and are more engaged in preventive programmes, which favours the maintenance of physical and organic integrity (SZE et al., 2008; MACHADO et al., 2011).

The data obtained in the study shows polypharmacy and the concomitant use of various medicines. The greater number of comorbidities makes the use of polypharmacy frequent among the elderly. Higher consumption was found in the study by Sze et al. in which, of the 56 community-dwelling elderly people who took part in the sample, 50 per cent used three or more medicines. The concomitant use of several drugs increases the likelihood of drug interaction and adverse reactions that can lead to postural hypotension and alterations in the central nervous system, resulting in disturbances in vision, proprioception, balance and coordination.

The prevalence of falls of 53.6% found in this study was higher than the data shown in the national (PINHO et al., 2012; BEKIBELE, 2010) and international literature (MILAT et al., 2011; HALIL et al., 2006), however, this result can be compared to the research carried out by Fabrício (2004) and Lopes (2009), in which, respectively, 54% and 54.4% of elderly Brazilians living in communities fell.

Population studies carried out in Brazil have recorded variations in the prevalence of falls, which is more pronounced when it comes to recurrent falls, especially when comparing Western and Eastern countries, which have a percentage almost double that of Western countries (CHU 2005; SALVÀ, 2004).

In our research, the data follows the alarming statistics from Eastern countries and exceeds the findings in the national literature, since 27.8 per cent said they had fallen twice or more, pointing to the need for local preventive strategies and policies (SANTER et al., 2012).

The higher occurrence of falls in women corroborates other studies that relate the fact that women are more fragile, have a higher prevalence of chronic diseases and are exposed to domestic activities that can pose a risk (FHON et al., 2012; PEREIRA et al., 2013).

Unlike studies that have shown an association between age and falls in this study, although the event was higher among older people (56 per cent of those over 69), the multivariate analysis showed no association between these variables (SIQUEIRA, 2007; CHU, 2005).

The elderly in our study were independent, active in the community, and the majority (73.5%) worked outside the home, which may have had some influence on this result.

Among the self-reported diagnoses, osteoarticular diseases maintained a significant association with a single fall event after the adjusted analysis, in line with what has been described in the literature (SACHETTI et al, 2010; MILATT, et. al, 2011).

Bekibeli and Gureje (2010), in a study of 2,090 elderly people, showed that the likelihood of osteoarticular diseases resulting in a fall is high, with rheumatoid arthritis increasing the chance of this almost twofold, which can be explained by the impairment in gait reaction time, coordination and balance resulting from joint pain.

Functional balance is widely assessed by the BBS, which was considered in some studies to be the instrument that best predicted the risk of falls in community-dwelling elderly people. In our study, lower performance on the BBS showed a positive association with the occurrence ($p < 0.01$) and recurrence of falls ($p = 0.03$) after multivariate analysis (SHUMWAY - COOK A, 2003; WHITNEY, 1999).

Shumway-Cook and collaborators (1997) found an association between injury and a low BSE score. These authors suggest that the test is the best single predictor of falls, with a non-linear relationship between the score and the risk of falling. Each point less increases the risk, and between scores 56 and 54, each point less is associated with a 3 to 4 per cent increase in the chance of falling. From 54 to 46, a change of one point increases the risk by 6 to 8 per cent, while below 36 points, the chance of falling is 100 per cent.

Other studies have also found a risk of falling in community-dwelling elderly people assessed by the BSE. One way of increasing functional balance and reducing the risk of falling is to practise physical activity. Multimodal physical training involving aerobic exercise, strength, power, flexibility, coordination and balance is effective for this purpose (DONAT, ÖZCAN, 2007; GILLESPIE, 2009).

Although the occurrence of one or more falls was higher among sedentary elderly people (87.3% and 72.6% respectively), in this study there was no association between these variables. Despite this, this data deserves attention since inactivity predisposes to frailty, disability and mortality, and is considered a target of concern in preventive actions developed within the scope of primary care (GÓMES-CONESA, 2008).

As it is a multifactorial condition, the risk of falling and recurrent falls increases linearly with the number of risk factors. Tinetti et al. (1998) showed that there is an 8 per cent chance of the elderly with no risk falling and a 78 per cent chance for those with four or more factors. Sai et al. (2010) also showed an association between the number of risk variables and recurrent falls, since those who had only one fall had fewer risk factors than those who had fallen 2 or more times.

In our study, the physical performance measures of elderly people with recurrent falls were lower than those who fell only once, with a statistically significant difference in all the clinical tests used. However, apart from the BSE, the variables that remained in the final model and were associated with the recurrence of falls were the TUG and the FES-I.

The time taken to perform the TUG is recognised as important in the literature and when it is over 12 seconds, it characterises the elderly person as being at high risk (STEFFEN, 2002*)*. The association between the TUG and a single fall described in other studies was not found in this study (THRANE, 2007). Similar to this result, Sain (2010) showed no difference in the test between elderly people who fell and those who didn't, but found that it was a predictor of two or more falls. This highlights the importance of gait in identifying recurrent falls, suggesting that prevention programmes involve activities aimed at training this variable.

Fear of falling was described by those who had suffered one, two or more episodes, and this variable was only associated with recurrent falls.

Low self-confidence in avoiding falls is an independent risk factor for disability and reduced mobility. It is also related to a decline in functionality, increased frailty, depression, anxiety and loss of social contact, all of which have repercussions on balance (BROUWER et al., 2003). According to Morris et al. (2004), elderly people who have suffered recurrent falls are more afraid of falling than those who have fallen only once, which may explain the association found in our study.

Most elderly people develop a fear of falling again after suffering a fall with serious consequences, resulting in greater restriction of activities and mobility, with a consequent cumulative increase in functional impairment in the prediction of recurrent falls.

The results of this study should be seen in the light of some limitations, such as sample loss, which may be associated with the fact that data collection was carried out on the premises of the BHU, which may have discouraged the participation of those who, for whatever reason, have difficulties with transport or are unavailable or unmotivated to attend events held at the BHU. This fact also made it impossible to assess home risks and approach the location of the fall, which are important in a study on this condition.

It is important to emphasise the possibility of respondent bias in relation to the occurrence of falls, since the elderly may have omitted the event due to forgetfulness, shame or fear, suggesting the relevance of follow-up studies addressing the elderly in the context of UBS.

A second issue concerns the cross-sectional design, which makes it impossible to verify causal associations between variables. Furthermore, the bivariate analysis prevents consideration of the possible confounding factors that permeate the determination of falls in the sample studied. In this way, it is important to highlight that this study aimed to identify the set of variables that best contribute to identifying the probabilistic occurrence of falls and recurrent falls, helping to identify risk factors that are easily identifiable by health professionals, which allows for a quick and effective approach that can reduce their occurrence, benefiting the elderly, their carers and the health system itself.

REFERENCES

Almeida APPV de, Veras RP, Doimo LA. Evaluation of the static and dynamic balance of elderly women practising water aerobics and gymnastics. **Revista Brasileira de Cineantropometria e Desenvolvimento Humano** 2010; 12(1):55- 61.

Alves NB, Scheicher ME. Postural balance and risk of falling in elderly people in the city of Garça, SP. ***Rev Bras Geriatr Gerontol 2011***; 14(4): 763 - 768.

Bekibele CO, Gureje O. Fall incidence in a population of elderly persons in Nigeria. ***Gerontology*** 2010; 56(3):278-283.

Berg KO, Wood-Dauphinee SL, Williams JI, Maki B. Measuring balance in the elderly: validation of an instrument. **Canadian Journal of Public** Health 1992; 83: 7- 11.

Bertakis KD, Azari R, Helms LJ,Callahan EJ, Robbins JA. Gender Differences in the Utilisation of Health Care Services. **The Journal of Family Practice** 2000; 49 (2): 147- 152.

Bertollucci PHF, Brucki SMD, Campacci SR, et al. The mini-mental state examination in a general population: impact of schooling. ***Arq*** *Neurol* 1994; 52(1): 1-7.

Brouwer BJ, Walker C, Rydahl SJ, Culham EG. Reducing fear of falling in seniors through education and activity programmes: a randomized trial. ***J Am Geriatr So.*** 2003;51(6): 829 - 834.

Camargos FOO, Dias RC, Dias JMD, Freire MTF. Cross-cultural adaptation and evaluation of the psychometric properties of the Falls Efficacy Scale - International in elderly Brazilians (FES - I- Brazil). ***Rev. Bras. Fisioter*** 2010; 14(3): 237 - 243.

Chu LW, Chi I, Chiu AY. Incidence and predictors of falls in the chinese elderly. ***Ann Acad Med Singap*** 2005; 34(1): 60 - 72.

Cruz DT, Ribeiro LC, Vieira MT, Texeira MTB, Bastos RR, Leite ICG. Prevalence of falls and associated factors. ***Rev Saude Publica*** 2012; 46(1).

Cruz, D. T.; Leite, I. C. G. Rev. Brasil. Geria. Geront. Falls and associated factors in community-dwelling elderly. 2018, n. 21, v. 5.

Dantas EL, de Brito GEG, Lobato IAF. Prevalence of falls in elderly people enrolled in the Family Health Strategy in the municipality of João Pessoa, Paraíba. ***Rev APS*** 2012; 15(1): 67 - 75.

Donat H, Özcan A. Comparison of the effectiveness of two programmes on older adults at risk of falling: unsupervised home exercise and supervised group exercise. ***Clinic Rehabil*** 2007; 21: 273-283.

Ecorsim, S. M. Ageing in Brazil: social, political and demographic aspects analysed
Serv. Soc. Soc., 2021. n. 141, p. 427- 446.

Ekezie JCK, Onwukamuche GE, Ugochukwu AI. Incidence of Fall Related Hip Fractures among the Elderly Persons in Owerri, Nigeria. Asian Journal of Medical Sciences 2011; 3(3): 110-114.

.

Fhon JRS, Wehbe SCCF, Vendruscolo TRP, Stackfleth R, Marques S, Rodrigues RAP. Falls in the elderly and their relationship with functional capacity. ***Rev. Latino- Am. Enfermagem*** 2012: 20(5).

Gillespie LD, Robestson MC, Gillespie WJ et al. Interventions for preventing falls in older people living in the community. **Cochrane Database of Syst Rev** 2009; 4(6): 1-193.

Gai J, Gomes L, Nóbrega OT de, Rodrigues MP. Factors associated with falls in community-dwelling elderly women. Journal of the Brazilian Medical Association 2010; 56 (3): 327-32.

.

Gómes-Conesa A, Gama ZAS. Risk factors for falls in the elderly: a systematic review. **Rev Saude Publica** 2008; 42(5): 946 - 956.

Ganança FF, Gazzola JM, Aratani MC, Perracini MR, Ganança MM. Circumstances and consequences of falls in elderly people with chronic vestibulopathy. **Brazilian Journal of Otorhinolaryngology** 2006(3).

GONÇALVES, I. C. M. Trends in mortality due to falls in the elderly in Brazil between 2000 and 2019. **Rev. Bras. Epidemiol** 2022; n 25.

Halil M, Ulger Z, Cankurtaran M, Shorbagi A, Yavuz BB, Dede D, Ozkayar N, Ariogul S. Falls and the elderly: is there any difference in the developing world? A cross-sectional study from Turkey. ***Arch Gerontol Geriatr*** 2006; 43(3): 351-359

Laboissière P. Agência Brasil. Available at: [accessed 2010 Sep 1] **Available** at: http://agenciabrasil.ebc.com.br/saude/journal_content/56/19523/1066161.

Lopes KT, Costa DP, Santos LP, Castro DP, Bastone AC. Prevalence of fear of falling in a community-dwelling elderly population and its correlation with mobility, dynamic balance, risk and history of falls. Revista Brasileira de Fisioterapia 2009; 13(3): 223-229.

Lin M, Hwang H, Wang Y, Chang S, Wolf SL. Community-based Tai Chi and its effect on injurious falls, balance, gait, and fear of falling in older people. Physical Therapy 2006; 86(9): 1189-1202.

Maciel ACC, Guerra RO. Prevalence and factors associated with balance deficit in the elderly. Revista Brasileira de Ciência e Movimento 2005; 13 (1): 37-44.

Machado JC, Ribeiro RCL de, Cotta RMM, Leal PFG da. Cognitive decline in the elderly and its association with epidemiological factors in Viçosa, Minas Gerais. **Brazilian Journal of Geriatrics and Gerontology** 2011; 14(1).

Milat AJ, Watson WL, Monger C, Barr M, Giffin M, Reid M. Prevalence, circumstances and consequences of falls among community-dwelling older people: results of the 2009 NSW Falls Prevention Baseline Survey. ***NSW Public Health Bulletin*** 2011; 22(3-4): 60 - 68.

Miyamoto ST, Lombardi JI, Berg KO et al. Brazilian version of the Berg balance scale. ***Braz J Med Biol Res*** 2004; 37 (9): 1411-1421.

MORRIS, M, Osborne D, Hill K, Kendig H, Lundgren- Lindquist B, Browning C, Reid J. Predisposing factors for occasional and multiple falls in older Australians who live at home. Aust J **Physiother** 2004; 50(3): 153-159.

Nascimento FA, Vareschi AP, Alfieri FM. Prevalence of falls, associated factors and functional mobility in institutionalised elderly people. **Arquivos Catarinenses de Medicina** 2008; 37(2): 7- 12.

Paiva, M. M; Lima, M. G.; Barros, M. B. A. **Social inequalities in the impact of falls among the elderly on health-related quality of life.** Rev. Ciência e Saúde Coletiva 2020; n. 25, v. 5.

Pereira AA, Ceolim MF, Neri AL. Association between insomnia symptoms, daytime napping and falls in community-dwelling elderly. **Cad Saude Publica** 2013: 29(3): 535 - 546.

Piovesan AC, Pivetta HMF, Peixoto JMB de. Factors predisposing to falls in elderly residents in the western region of Santa Maria, RS. Brazilian Journal of Geriatrics and Gerontology 2011; 14(1): 75- 83.

Pinho TAM, Silva AO, Turas LFR, Moreira MASP, Gurgels SN, Smiths AAF, Bezerra VP. Assessment of the risk of falls in elderly people attending a Basic Health Unit. ***Rev Esc Enf USP*** 2012; 46(12): 320 - 327.

Podsiadlo D, Richardson S. The timed Up & Go: A test of basic functional mobility for frail elderly persons. ***J Am Geriatr Soc*** 1991; 39(2): 142-148.

Rozenfeld S. Prevalence, associated factors and medication misuse among the elderly: a review. **Cadernos de Saúde Pública** 2003;

Rubenstein LZ. Falls in older people: epidemiology, risk factors and strategies for prevention. **Age and Aging** 2006; 35: 37-41.

Sachetti A, Vidmar MF, da Silveira MM, Schneider RH, Wibelinger LM. Risk of falling in elderly people with osteoporosis. **Rev Bras Cienc Saude** 2010: 8(24): 23 - 25.

Sai AJ, Gallagher JC, Smith LM, Logsdon S. Fall predictors in the community dwelling elderly:A cross sectional and prospective cohort study. **J Musculoskelet Neuronal Interact** 2010; 10(2): 142 - 150.

Salvà A, Bolíbar I, Pera G, Arias C. Incidence and consequences of falls among elderly people living in the community. ***Med Clin*** 2004; 122(5): 172 - 176.

Santer T, Bruggemann CFVP, da Silva OM. Prevalence of falls among elderly people attending basic health units in the municipality of Palmitos, Santa *Catarina, and associated factors.* ***Rev Saude Publica*** *2012; 5(2): 32 - 43.*

Shumway-cook A, Brauer S, Woollacott MH. Predicting the Probability for Falls in Community-Dwelling Older Adults Using The Timed Up & Go Test. Physical Therapy 2000: 80(9): 896- 903.

Shumway-Cook A, Brauer S, Woollacott MH. Predicting the Probability for Falls in Community-Dwelling Older Adults Using The Timed Up & Go Test. ***Phys Ther*** 2000; 80(9): 896- 903.

Silsupadol P, Shumway-Cook A, Lugade V et al. Effects of Single-Task Versus Dual-Task Training on Balance Performance in Older Adults: A Double-Blind, Randomised Controlled Trial. Archives of Physical Medicine and Rehabilitation. 2009; 90(3): 381-387.

Sze P, Cheung W, Lam P, Dominic H, Leung K, Chan T. The Efficacy of a Multidisciplinary Falls Prevention Clinic With an Extended Step-Down Community Programme. Archives of Physical Medicine and Rehabilitation 2008; 80: 1329- 1334.

Steffen TM, Hacker TA, Mollinger L. Age- and gender-related test performance in community-dwelling elderly people: Six-Minute Walk Test, Berg Balance Scale, Timed Up & Go Test, and gait speeds. **Phys Ther** 2002; 82(2): 128 - 137.

Thrane G, Joakimsen RM, Thornquist E. The association between timed up and go test and history of falls: The tromso study. **BMC Geriatr** 2007;7(1): 1 - 7

Tinetti ME, Williams CS. The effect of falls and falls injuries on functioning in community-dwelling older persons. ***J Gerontol*** 1998; 53(2): 429 - 434.

Whitney SL, Poole JL, Cass SP. A review of balance instruments for older adults. The American Journal of Occupational Therapy 1998; 53 (8): 666-671.

Yardley L, Beyer N, Klaus H. Development and initial validation of the Falls Efficacy Scale-International (FES-I); Age and Ageing 2005; 34: 614-619.

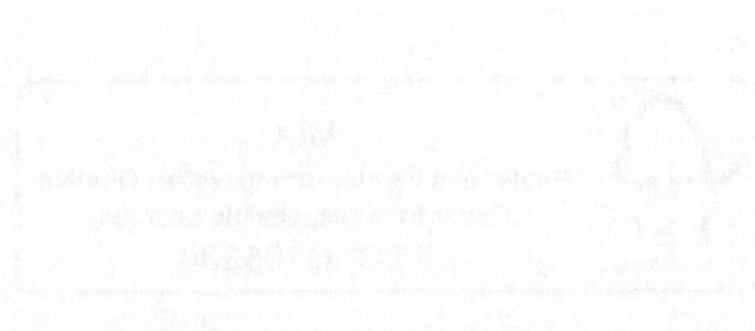

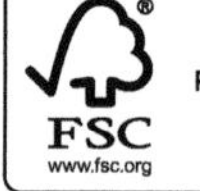

MIX
Papier aus verantwortungsvollen Quellen
Paper from responsible sources
FSC® C105338

Printed by Books on Demand GmbH, Norderstedt / Germany